The Skinny Dragon
Plan- Basic

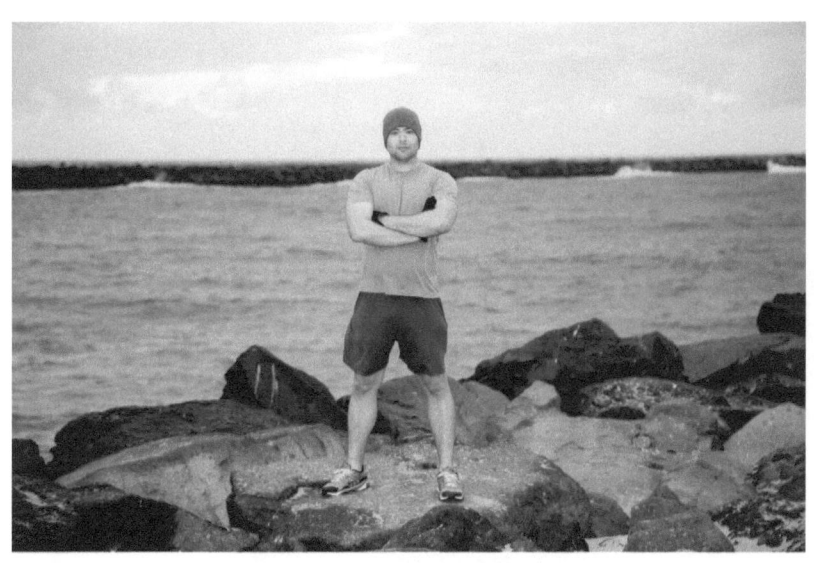

Dr. Robert Lee Garcia

**While this book may be offensive to some, it's written with the desire to help others have the lifestyle of their dreams. I have been an overweight person for over half my life and the change in attitude after weight loss literally made me a new person. If any content stings a little, its because I love you and want to see you succeed - Dr. Garcia

Table of Contents

All information used in this book utilizing outside sources were gathered in strict compliance with the Fair Use Act for the purposes of education and research. 17 USC § 107.

NOTE: Dr. Robert Garcia is not a Medical Doctor. He has an Ed.D, which is the Educational version of a Ph.D. He has no nutritional training and has never been to Med School. He HAS, however, researched everything in this book and personally uses the Skinny Dragon Plan to manage his weight.

he is in a joint operations combat unit in the military, has done a 16 mile, nonstop beach run for fun, and is a columnist for Fitness Inked magazine. Who would you rather listen to, some skinny, geeky medical school flunky that will tell you to live on salads, or a guy that loves Coors light and chasing Hooters waitresses?

Dr. Rob Garcia assumes no responsibility for the results

gained from this plan. The liability lies strictly on the user.

Dr. Rob Garcia cannot be responsible when you have to throw out your old clothes because they don't fit, or if you start getting looks from the opposite sex that are far more than friendly. He would absolutely hate it if your friends and family started worrying about you because you dropped 10 pounds in less than two weeks.

Embrace the plan at your own risk... of awesomeness.

Dr. Rob Garcia

Skinny Dragon Plan- Basic

1. Intro

Imagine a bright Monday morning. You are in the kitchen getting the kids ready for school. Your son, Jimmy, walks to the kitchen table and sits down. You make him a bowl of cereal and pour bleach over it. While he is eating it, you prepare his lunch, a bag of rat poison pellets, a carton of antifreeze, and then a nice bottle of Drano.

Sound dramatic? It should. This is exactly what millions of Americans are doing to themselves everyday when they make their meals. You wouldn't feed yourself and your family poison, would you? But you are. Every day you embrace a white flour and sugar filled confectionary lifestyle, you are adding to your waistline, increasing your chance for obesity related disease, and teaching your children bad habits from an early age.

I am here to teach you about how to eat properly. This plan will not only guide you to a better way of eating, it will help you to *a better life*. It will use these magical concepts like portion control, avoidance of high sodium foods, reduction of flour, and accelerated digestion. I know that for many of us, the battle for weight management is a long fought and slow to win war that never seems to end and if you are like me, you have at least two friends that can eat anything and never gain a pound, while you have a "fun size" bag of Wheat Thins and pop a button on your pants.

Practiced properly, this plan will not only teach you to eat properly, but at the right times. After a while, *it becomes easier to manage*.

My personal plan involves a lot more discipline. I have outlined it in my second book in this series, **The Skinny Dragon Plan- Advanced**. Once you master the concepts that are summarized in this book, pick up the Advanced plan and REALLY see what food management is about. There are tricks in there that you will swear are concocted by Satan.

This book is broken down into several sections that serve to not only teach you about nutrition, but to teach you WHY we get fat and how our parents contributed to this problem (we still love our parents, but they could definitely use this plan). I'll start off by telling you how awesome I am, and the steps that got me to write this book, the history of agriculture and how it added to obesity rates, how flour became the 'white devil' of nutrition, and much more. I'll also tell you how I created this plan by reverse engineering several of the most popular diet plans out there today.

My goal for you is to have you experience several enlightening moments such as:

*Losing enough weight so that your spouse/significant other gets "THAT" look in their eyes when they see you.

*Being able to throw out your regular clothes because they don't fit anymore.

*Walking down the street and getting eyes from the opposite sex (or the same sex, if that's your thing, I'm not judging you, playboy).

*Running into your ex and their new love interest and giving them a smirk and a wave.

*Being able to get up in the morning, look in the mirror and feel AMAZING about your progress.

I have experienced all of these things, and trust me, It's better than chocolate covered crack. There is NO greater feeling than knowing that you have results to show from your sacrifice.

2. Dr. Rob Garcia's Bio

Before you begin this plan, I want to tell you a little about myself so you understand where I am coming from. I want you to know that under all the trash talking, the confidence, and the possible hate mail I may receive from this book, is a genuinely compassionate person that *just wants you to be happy*. I didn't write this to become rich, I wrote it to give you a better life, if you so desire.

I was raised in a small logging town called Eureka, California. We didn't have a lot of money in our family, and not to call anyone out, but obesity runs in our genetics. I was a chubby kid, and it affected my self esteem, my friendships, and kept me from having the confidence to have a girlfriend in high school. My mom was a cook and my grandmother was Southern. My other grandmother owned Mexican restaurants. Obesity wasn't discussed, but it was the elephant in the room, so to speak.

As I grew up, I was a pudgy teen and started skateboarding. It helped but wasn't a perfect solution. Finally I left town, and eventually joined the Air Force. The PT and then learning about working out helped me to get muscular but not fit. I still didn't understand nutrition or the need to eat correctly.

I moved to San Diego in 2002. I was still a slightly chubby adult. One day, I was in the library and by accident found a book written by a guy in his 70s. He had been heavy his whole life, and one day gave up flour and started eating watermelon. He lost a bunch of weight rapidly and took up ballroom dancing! That book (for the life of me, I can't remember its name) changed my perspective on things. I embraced the "no flour" movement and around the same time, several of my friends were having great results with the Atkins Diet.

I had a SIGNIFICANT weight loss and was doing pretty well for a few years. I joined the reserves and had an annual PT test which became every six months if you don't score a

90 or above. I started a very intense exercise regimen and incorporated running as a staple of my cardio plan. I still fluctuated here and there. I created a meal plan and put it on my blog, The Blue Dragon Enterprises Blog, around 2010. A few people tried it and had good results. It incorporated small meals, reduction of flour, and contained a floor workout for toning the body.

Around October of 2013, a few things happened. I read several amazing books that changed my perspective, and I finally took my buddy's advice. On October 19th, I was awarded my Ed.D in Education. I started tripling the amount of reading I did, and I hit the mother load.

I read *Man 2.0: Engineering The Alpha*, and Tim Ferriss' *4 Hour Body*. First of all, I would STRONGLY suggest getting these books. After I read them, I started reading and learning about the top diet plans in the country. Atkins, Paleo, The Zone, South Beach. I reverse engineered all of them, and figured out the essential components and the hows and whys of their effectiveness.

The end result? The Skinny Dragon Diet. A plan that I GAVE away to a test group of friends. The results amazed even me. Some quotes:

> *"I lost 10 pounds in a week. I got my mom on it too."*
>
> *"My friends say I am glowing. I can't wait to buy new clothes."*
>
> *"You are onto something BIG. And contagious. All my friends want to try it."*

After seeing these successes, I decided to take the plunge and write this book. I have happily used the plan, although a lot stricter than my friends, and my results have been great. More muscle, faster fat loss, a cheat day, and better fitting clothes.

I believe in this plan. As must you. If you can make the initial commitment to following its rules, a new life awaits you.

3. No Excuses

This chapter may come across as harsh, but it needs to be written. Anyone that uses this plan will need to erase all doubt. It has become easier to just "go with the flow" and accept being at an unsafe and unhealthy weight. The movement to call women of a certain size BBWs, the popularity of Lane Bryant stores, and enormous portions in fast food and restaurants have created this perfect storm of fat acceptance. You must NOT buy into this.

On the flip side, I do NOT advocate "fat shaming." I feel that everyone deserves to be happy, healthy, and not feel like a goddamn pariah because they are having trouble with managing a good weight for their lifestyle.

I was particularly intrigued by Maria Kang, the "fit mom" who posted a picture of her in gym attire with a heading that said "What's your excuse?" while surrounded by her three young children. The backlash from moms was overwhelming. They thought she was fat shaming them, and to be honest, many were probably jealous because she bounced back so quickly (and looked hot in the process).

It created a firestorm of controversy, with many applauding her, and many hating her. She handled it with class. I don't see her putting down other moms, I see her as issuing a challenge- "I did it, so can you." Good for her. The only people that would have an issue with that are whining losers that hate their lives. Maria didn't talk down to anyone, in fact, she showed initiative, and did not use childbirth as an excuse for obesity.

I struggle with my weight daily. DAILY. I must take aggressive steps to keep at a certain level of fitness. This means frequent 6 mile plus runs, gym visits at 5 am, NO weekly desserts or lunches with coworkers, and carrying my own food like a refugee to work everyday. It takes discipline because my body is slow to respond and really, really likes chocolate and red velvet cake.

I have dealt firsthand with the reactions of people when you are overweight. It affects every aspect of your life, believe it or not: dating, employment, everything. This is why I feel so strongly about the subject. I will not sympathetically hold your hand, and tell you that "you are beautiful just how you are" and advocate bad eating habits. I won't let you raise your kids to be obese. I get infuriated when I see a large woman with three obese kids and they are buying nothing but flavored sugar water, white bread, chips, and cookies.

Have you ever used any of these excuses? (I have)

*Fat runs in my family. I just have to accept it.
*I have a thyroid issue.
*I just love desserts too much.
*My spouse likes me with a little extra meat.
*I'm too tired to prepare or cook my food.
*It's easier to eat out.
*I'm supposed to keep some baby weight after childbirth.

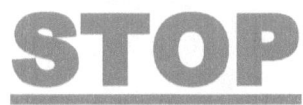

Most of these do not contain relevance to a problem with obesity. I was a good excuse maker for many years. The only problem that I had was a lack of discipline. I let my friends dictate many of my dietary choices, I was too lazy to pay attention to portion control, and I figured that since I had a few larger relatives, that I had to accept being large too.

I was wrong, and so are you if you buy into these excuses. First of all, thyroid conditions are often used as a crutch for everything. The last girl I dated blamed her obesity on thyroid issues, but had never been diagnosed. She also ate cake and cookies a few times a week, and drank often. It's too easy to have a vague, generic excuse when the real problem is your food routine. We didn't last long because she was an excuse maker, and wouldn't address the issue or stick to her goals.

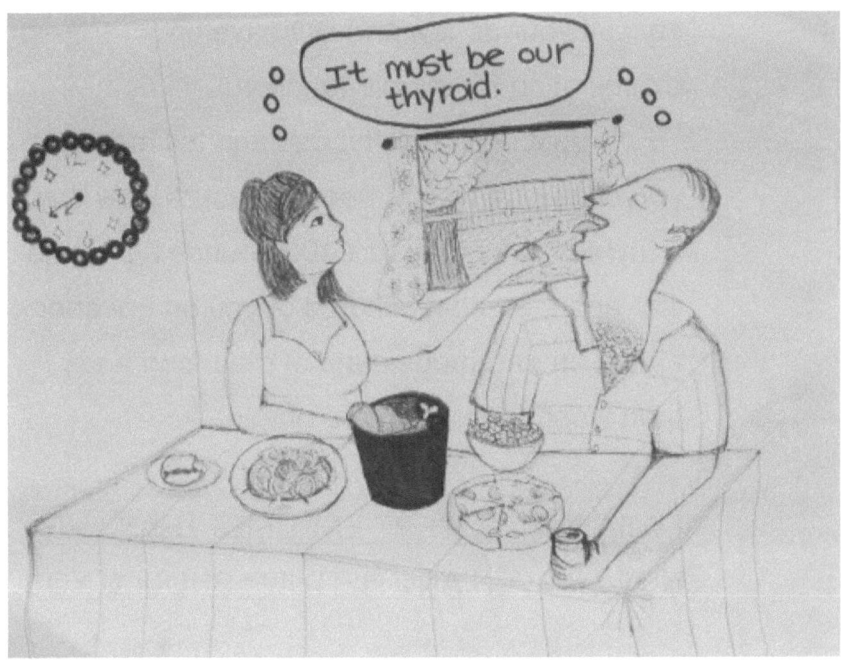

Just to be clear, some of us DO have medical issues, or mobility problems. I am not chastising you. Some of you will have chronic pain. I am not trying to make light of your situation. I just don't want others to use certain conditions as their crutch to avoid the real task of changing their eating routines.

Any person that uses this plan, follows it, and then incorporates regular exercise SHOULD see tangible results. If you do not see results after 30 days, I would tell you to consult your doctor and DO have an examination for thyroid function.

Just don't bullshit me, and tell me that you can't lose weight because your uncle "had a thyroid issue and was 400 pounds his whole life" and then post pictures of you on Facebook eating an enormous plate of fried food and then wonder why you are obese.

<u>I WILL NOT ACCEPT EXCUSES THAT ARE NOT PROVEN AND NEITHER SHOULD YOU.</u>

Once again, sorry to sound harsh. I promise I'll be nice and polite throughout the rest of the book. Excuses just piss me off, because I made them, and I lived through years of obesity *because* I made them.

<u>Once the excuses went away, so did the weight.</u>

4. FDA Food Pyramid and Agriculture

In order to understand how we as a society embraced obesity (damn you, Sara Lee), we must look back to the evolution of food creation. If history isn't your thing, feel free to skip ahead, I won't be offended. I am one of those guys that likes to know cause and effect.

Our current obesity problem can be related to a series of variables that are in our face daily. The following illustration shows the point:

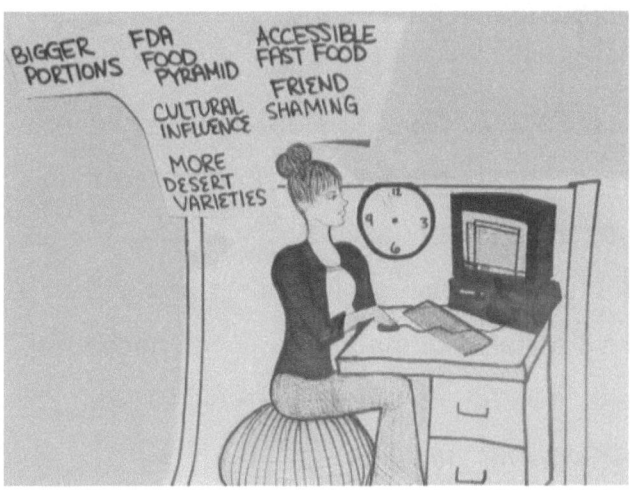

A person is deluged with all of these concepts and ideas about what a meal should consist of. Many are VERY harmful nutritionally. Some of these include:

1. Cultural- Certain traditional foods are not conducive to a healthy lifestyle. My African American friends tell me about family get togethers that have huge plates of chitlins, fried chicken, and ribs. My Polish friends are served beer and sausage. My own group, Hispanic, indulges in fried enchiladas, tacos, burritos, and breakfast is fried in lard.

2. Fast Food Access- Fast food is everywhere. It's fairly cheap, at nearly every corner and in some cases, even delivers. The sheer convenience is enough for most people to make it a staple of their diets. What people fail to realize is that fast food is a multi tiered attack on your waistline:

- High sodium content in the meat and fries makes you thirsty, and you consume soda
- Chemically altered to enhance flavor and cause addiction
- Deceptive marketing leads us to believe that low calories equals low sodium and fat content
- Deliberately targets children in order to drive them to crave it often
- Giant amount of empty calories from buns, bread, and fries

3. Parental Guilt- Remember the starving kids in China that were wasting away? The African children that would kill to have your brussel sprouts? The college freshmen wasting away in his dorm at Florida State because he paid for tuition instead of a basic meal plan? Neither do I. These were stupid things our parents told us to get us to eat. The problem is that most parents had a "clean your plate or no dessert" rule. This means that you were served a huge

portion of food, and had to shovel it down, THEN you got a sugar filled treat. No wonder most of us struggled with obesity as young people. Our parents, while meaning well, didn't understand about food groups, meal size, or nutritional research.

4. Friend Shaming- My coworkers should be beaten for this. How many times do you get invited to eat a 3,000 calorie lunch? For me, about 4 a week. Plus doughnuts in the morning. Plus holiday cake. Plus bagels. They are actually at the point where they leave treats on my desk to see if I will cave in. I have NEVER given in, not once. I respect them, I take their teasing every day with a smile, and I appreciate the camaraderie, but to be fit, you have to be master of your own destiny.

5. The Food Pyramid- My personal favorite. Remember this inaccurate, overused, piece of shit? (Sorry, I tend to speak my mind. Good for getting points across, bad for dating and job promotions).

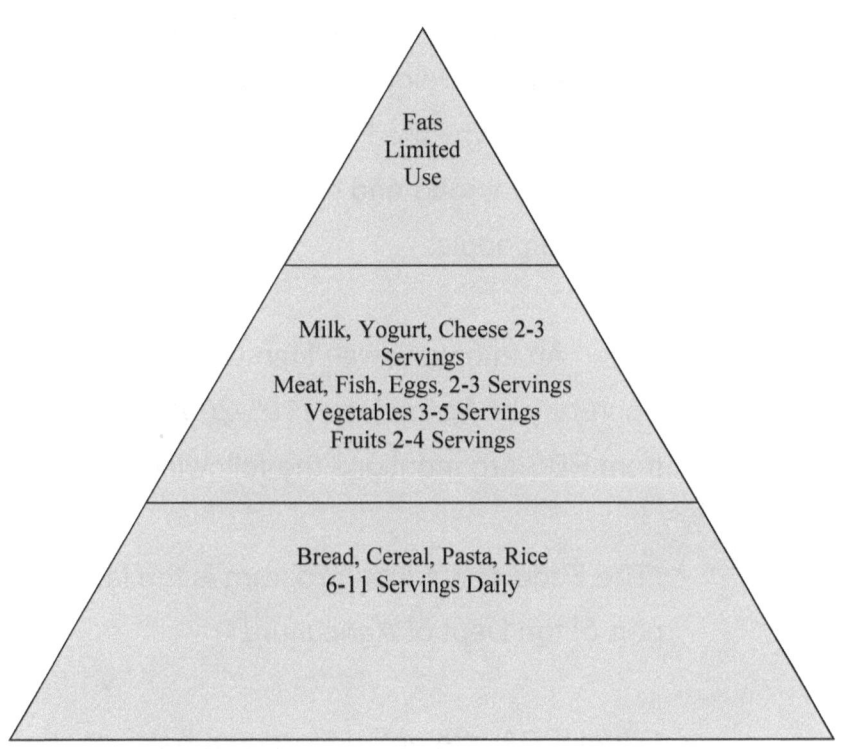

(I drew this. Don't be jealous)

Adults used this model shamelessly for my generation. I don't blame them. At the time, it seemed logical, balanced, and well thought out.

It was completely wrong. Let's examine this. I run about 20 miles a week. If I ate 11 servings of grain, rice, and pasta, every day, I'd look like Dom Delouise. I did some research and here is why the Food Pyramid is completely wrong and contributed to a nation of obese people.

An Interview with Dan Glickman, Secretary of Agriculture 1995-2001, retrieved from PBS.org mentions the following:

*The Federal nutrition program is the largest part of the Dept of Agriculture

*The USDA attempted to draw a balance between farmers and low income women and children

*When the Food Pyramid was created, the governing thought was that fats were bad and carbohydrates were good

The former Secretary of Agriculture has gone on record stating that:

1. The pyramid has too many carbohydrates.

2. The government overreacted in its promotion to push US grown products like dairy, meat, and grain, without data proving its healthiness.

3. The majority of the information on the pyramid was created to support government programs to feed low income women, infants, and food stamp recipients.

4. There is new research differentiating between good and bad fats, and whole grains vs. regular grains.

Let's get a second opinion. On the same PBS.org website is an interview with Walter Willet, M.D., the Chair at Harvard School of Public Health.
He states the following points:

*The food guide developed in 1991 implies that fats are bad, so that carbohydrates must be a better choice

*The Pyramid displays that we can eat 11 servings a day, plus potatoes are counted as a vegetable, so we can have 13 servings of starch a day

*It does not differentiate different types of fats and just tells us to reduce them

*It's been known for 40 years that the type of fat consumed was important. The pyramid was outdated immediately

*The dairy and beef industries were heavily represented in the pyramid

*Newer forms of the pyramid have incorporated weight control and regular activity, healthy fats are represented more

*The revised pyramids have red meat, dairy, and white breads, sweets, pasta and rice at the top suggesting that they should be minimally consumed

Dr. Willet suggests that there are far too many starches in the "Pyramid of Death" and that the type of fats that we are told to avoid have been known to be healthy for 40 years.

Dr. Willet, you have a sweet mustache, and unlike my Coors Light chugging ass, actually finished med school and made your family proud. You sound like a bro and I'd totally cruise Havasu with you while cranking some 'Tallica. Thanks for the supportive evidence.

I wanted to see what the other side of the spectrum had to say about the Food Pyramid so I started looking up athletes, real ones, not goofy dudes like me that watch Army Ranger videos and think we are badass because we run at 5 am with a Camelbak®.

Ben Greenfield, who is a nutritionist, a triathlete, and a holder of a Master's in Biomechanics and Exercise Physiology, offers this on his website, www.bengreenfieldfitness.com:

*Chinese and Greek food pyramids show high amounts of cereals, pasta, and grains

*This can lead to issues with health

*Studies have shown that healthy dietary fat has been proven to increase weight loss lowered blood sugar and shows normal brain functions in minors

*The recommendation of 2-4 servings of fruit is especially bad for your blood sugar

Here we have a triathlete with a Master's degree in Biomechanics and Exercise Physiology that fully supports my assertion that the Food Pyramid is worthless. Ben also looks a lot better than I do with his shirt off, so he should be trusted. Please go to his website, and buy some of his apparel or products. Ben has a great deal of knowledge and well written articles about fitness.

Skinny Dragon Plan- Basic

5. White Flour

Since aggressive limitation of flour is a key component of the Skinny Dragon Plan, I figured it should be necessary to tell you WHY flour is so damned bad for you. I researched Katheryn Mcgowan's blog about flour and its history. Here are some facts from her site:

This is a diagram of a wheat kernel.

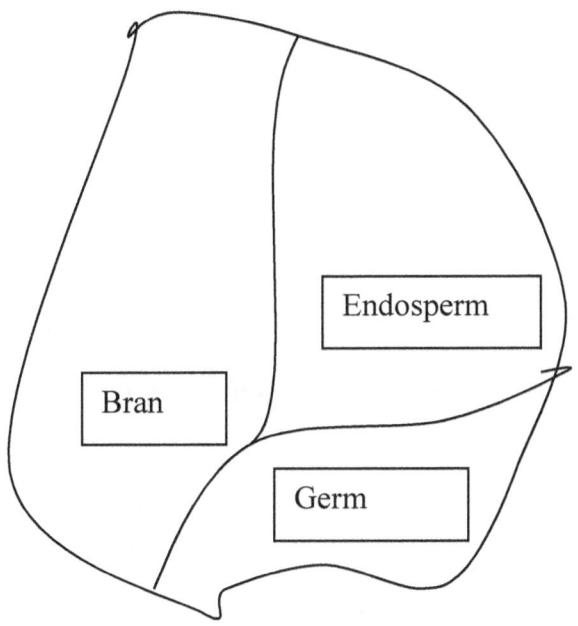

(Professional Illustration done by me with Microsoft Word Curvy Line)

All the nutrients are found in the bran and the germ. Between the two, they contain insoluble fiber, some B vitamins and Iron. The endosperm contains basic carbohydrates and minute amounts of nutrients.

The History

Back in ancient times, women would beat the kernel into flour using two rocks. This would have the effect of rupturing the germ, which would release wheat germ oil, and turn the flour a brownish color. Unfortunately, this process would also shorten the shelf life to about six months.

The process

Once industrial rollers came into play, flour could be created by stripping the kernel of the germ and bran. This had a duel effect. It doubled the shelf life of flour, and removed nearly all the nutrients from it. The access to longer lasting flour helped the population grow, but at the same time, contributed to several diseases that were caused by lack of nutritional value. During the 1930s, nutrients started being added to flour in order to stave off these ailments.

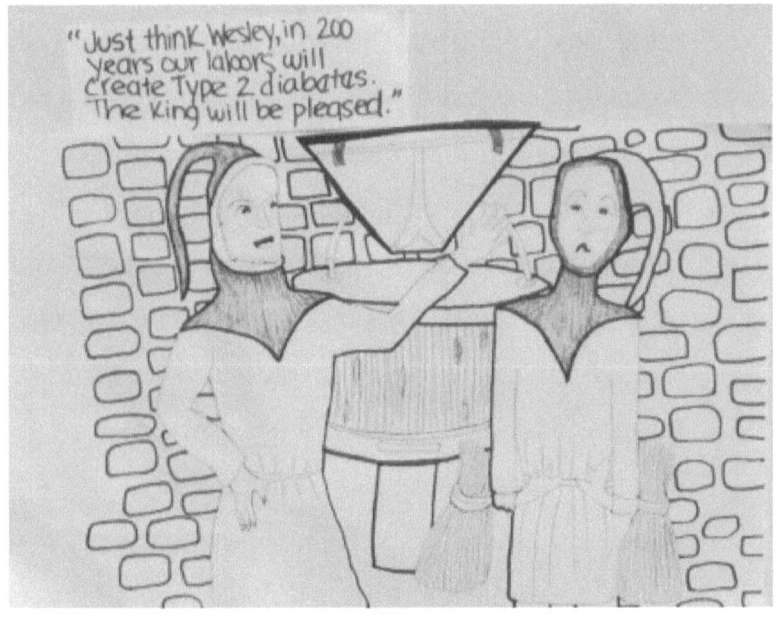

The Effect on Digestion

So what happens when you eat white flour? Why does Dr. Rob Garcia hate it so damn much? And why does red velvet cake taste like a gift from God? According to the website, www.care2.com, flour based foods are consumed in higher quantities because there is less chewing. Digestion occurs much faster with flour based goodies, and spikes your blood sugar. This in turn causes insulin to rise, which makes you hungry a few hours later, and increases your chance at diabetes if insulin resistance becomes a regularly occurring event.

In summary, eating flour causes you to be hungry faster, spikes your blood sugar, and inadvertently causes higher rates of consumption because it digests easily and doesn't need to be chewed as much. This is why I cannot eat Cheese Puff Cheetos. One goes in my mouth, and next thing I know, the bag is empty and I'm crying like I'm watching the Chargers lose to the Raiders.

The effect on Health

It doesn't stop there. Dr. Simon Dankel was recently interviewed about the relationship between type 2 diabetes and obesity. A researcher from Norway, that is in the United States for a year to study obesity related illnesses, he sheds light on this topic. From the kpcnews.com website, Dr. Dankel makes a few key points:

*Harvard provided a great opportunity to study specific genes that appear to be involved with Type 2 diabetes

*Diabetes has risen in the last 30 years and will continue to rise due to the increase in obesity

*To prevent diabetes, eat whole unrefined ingredients such as fresh fruits and vegetables and whole grain products

*Combining good diet and more exercise will reverse obesity and will promote well being

*In my opinion, the primary cause of Type 2 Diabetes is overeating refined carbohydrates (products made with white flour and sugar)

*Include quality fats like olive, canola oil and butter

We now have the recommendation of a man possessing a doctorate in nutrition and is studying at Harvard. That's a pretty damn smart guy.

Inflammation

Another factor that must be considered is inflammation. I was not aware of this condition until I started researching this book. A leading heart surgeon in Arizona, Dr. Dwight Lundell, wrote a great article about inflammation. Dr. Lundell is quite experienced. I believe strongly that his theories and concepts are sound. Not to mention that he has done or been a part of over 5.000 open heart surgeries.

To sum up his key points:
1. Use olive oil, not sunflower or corn oil so that you can reduce inflammation within your body.
2. White flour and sugar based desserts are culprits in the process of chronic inflammation that can lead to heart disease.
3. Not all fats are bad.

I think you are starting to realize why I get pissed off when my coworkers bring in cinnamon rolls. I've done enough research to understand the short and long term effects of flour based desserts on the body.

So how do we fight inflammation? Dr. Weil M.D., has the following guide on his website, www.drweil.com:

*Consume soy as a source of protein
*Antioxidant supplements like Vitamin C and E
*2-4 cups of tea a day
*Cooked Asian mushrooms to increase immune function
*Dark chocolate as an antioxidant
*Brown rice, barley, steel cut oats, quinoa

Overall, I think that Dr. Weil has created an excellent guide. I only disagree with the soy products and the pasta during the week. Soy increases estrogen production in men. I already own Cher cds and have a copy of "The Notebook", so I need to be careful. Other than those two items, this is a great guide and follows most of the concepts of the Skinny Dragon Plan.

Dr. Weir has been on the cover of Time Magazine twice. That's pretty impressive. If I were ever on the cover of Time, I would probably be in handcuffs.

Crikey, that bloke gave us diabetes!

Let's examine it from another angle. Let's take a healthy population and see what happens when foreign settlers introduce white flour to them. Here's a hint: It sucks, bro.

According to the Better Health Channel in Australia, the early indigenous Aboriginals were a healthy culture of hunter/gatherers. They had no exposure to disease and lived strong and productive lives. Their diet was carbohydrates, nutrients, and protein.

As soon as flour, sugar, and processed meat were introduced to the population, the following diet-related diseases started affecting them heavily:

o Cardiovascular disease

o Diabetes

o Overweight and obesity

o High blood pressure

o Some cancers

o Circulatory diseases

o Stroke.

The Aboriginals were often paid in food. Their dietary consumption changed and their overall health declined. This should be a wakeup call to everyone that thinks that there are no effects from that bagel in the morning, pasta at lunch, and bread at night.

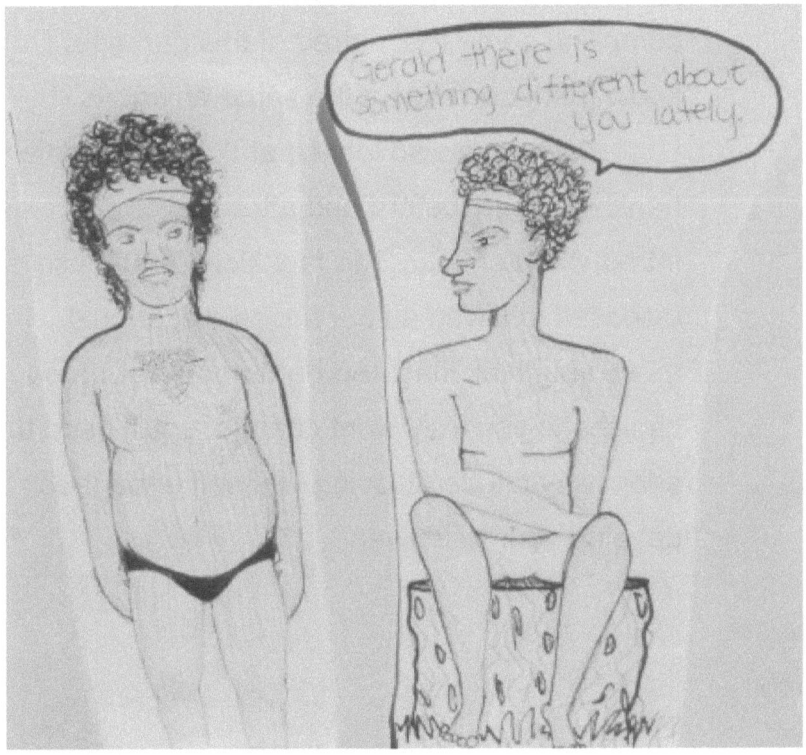

By now you guys are starting to get the picture. We have now read the opinions of three medical doctors, a triathlete, and learned about the effects of consumption of flour. We examined the process of how it is made, and the determinate factors of why it has barely any nutritional value. By now you should be compiling some real hatred of this garbage. I know that I don't see it the same anymore.

We have also looked at the effects on a healthy society before and after the introduction of flour. The fact alone that these diseases *followed* a flour based diet should make you think long and hard about your food choices. If you truly want change, you'll need to adopt an attitude of loving yourself enough to develop your willpower.

Let's be clear. I am NOT saying you should completely give up flour for the rest of your life and suffer when a coworker brings in cupcakes. In the Skinny Dragon Advanced Plan, you get a cheat day weekly, when you have moved along far enough in the Basic program. Cheat day means ANYTHING GOES. My cheat days are spent at Chilis.

For now, start to really think about the effects of a flour based food plan.

1. Increased appetite
2. Spiked blood sugar
3. Higher rates of obesity, and possibility of obesity-related disease such as heart disease, Type 2 diabetes, and high blood pressure
4. Feeling hungry soon after meals
5. Inflammation of your internal organs (proven to be a key factor in Alzheimer's, heart disease, and circulatory issues)

So I ask you, in all honesty, is that roll or muffin or cake, really worth it?

Skinny Dragon Plan- Basic

6. American Obesity Rates

Its time to face some ugly truths; We are now the second fattest industrialized nation in the world. According to the Huffington Post, Mexico barely beat us but we came in a close second. America now has an obesity rate of 31.8 percent. That's nearly one in three adults. It's interesting to note that a few things have occurred that helped Mexico to beat us. Heart disease and diabetes are killing Mexican adults faster than having to sit through a matinee of Madea movies.

Sugary foods and processed flour based foods are now a lot more plentiful and the poorest households have used these foods to edge out fresh fruits and vegetables (HuffPo, "Latino Politics"). Mexico is having the same issues we are, same introduction of low nutrition, high calorie food, and a skyrocketing of obesity, heart disease and diabetes.

I LOVE Mexican food. Especially California
burritos, but we need to make changes. We
can have our guacamole and eat it too. One
suggestion is using corn tortillas
instead of flour, and realizing that a full meal at
a Mexican restaurant is about three regular
sized meals. Remember, salsa is one of the
best things you can eat, and fills you up faster.
Avoid the fried stuff, and you should be ok.

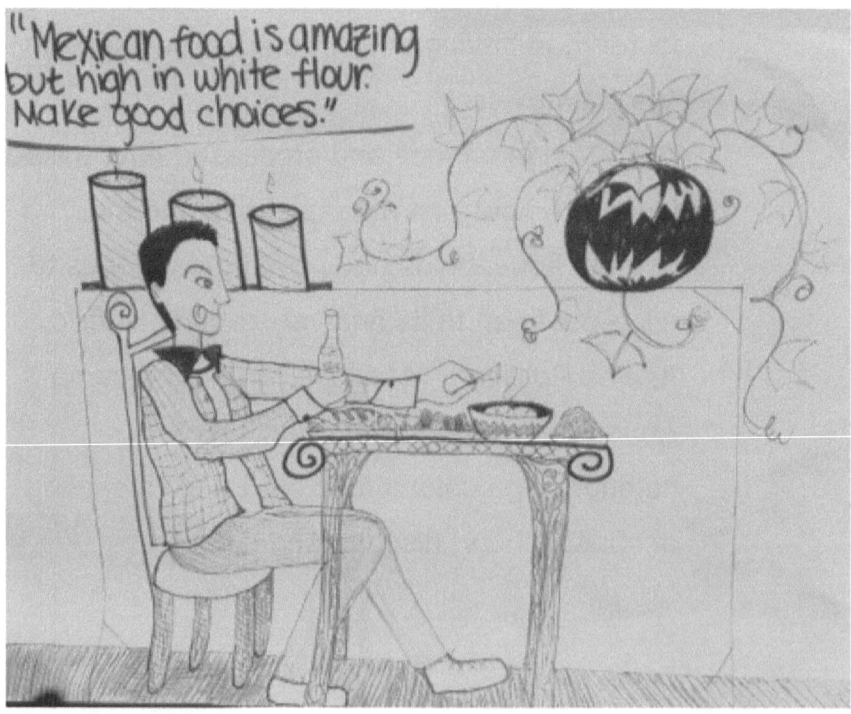

7. Medical Issues: Knees/Organs/Disease

I think it's important to point out a few facts related to disease and obesity. I know what you are thinking; is he ever going to get to the damn plan? Yes, but be patient. I have had to sit through a lot of things that I didn't feel were important. My date's stories about her hamster, Mr. Pickles, the Royal Wedding, the Sex in the City movie; this is educational, it won't kill you.

With obesity comes a host of damaging effects to the body. The worst part is that they start to create a circular effect. Once a person starts eating badly, they start exercising less. This causes fat gain. Their knees have to carry a higher load, which creates joint pain and eventually mobility issues. Once exercise and mobility decreases, even more weight is gained. Its a perfect storm for a sedentary lifestyle and a lifetime of soaps, bon bons, US Weekly and Oprah.

Don't do it. Don't accept it for a second, don't believe that things will magically get better "one day."

That day is TODAY.

Need some inspiration? If you have kids, imagine not being able to watch them grow up, missing their graduation or their wedding day, because you had no control, no willpower to streamline your life and your fitness. Acceptance of obesity is not just detrimental, it can be fatal.

According to a study by Oxford University researchers, moderately obese people live three years less , and severely obese live *ten* years less (than the average healthy person). It no longer is acceptable for Americans to be dying from a *preventable* condition. There is tremendous hope though.

According to a study that was published in the medical journal Lancet, "*Overweight and obese people could slash their increased risk of heart disease by half and their increased risk of stroke by three quarters by controlling their blood pressure, cholesterol and blood sugar*"

This is great news. By adopting a better diet, and monitoring your body's vital signs, you are extending your life. That is why I wrote this book, so I could see you in your 70s playing with your grandchildren, happy and healthy.

Fat Facts

According to the CDC, Type 2 diabetes is now affecting children more often. This is significant because it indicates a correlation with the lowering of nutritional standards for young children. I was also saddened to see that overweight children are now at risk for kidney problems, possible blindness and amputations.

It's time we stood up as Americans, and aggressively looked at this issue. No more excuses, no more silent acceptance. We don't need people losing limbs

because of bad nutrition and low willpower. This CAN be stopped.

Some interesting facts on the CDC website; Non Hispanic blacks are the most likely to be obese at nearly half, while Mexican Americans are at 40 percent. Educated women are less likely to be obese and Louisiana and Mississippi were the fattest states with over 30 percent of the population. (No more fried Twinkies at the fair, mister).

A study by the University of Rochester noted the following information:

1. Obese women are far more likely to develop severe knee problems as they get older.

2. Knee osteoarthritis is a serious condition that affects women in 70 percent of cases, particularly over 50.

3. Obesity is a modifiable factor in avoiding OA.

2. Every pound of weight lost may result in a four pound reduction in loads carried by the knee.

3. 5% weight loss results in 18% improvement in function.

These facts alone demonstrate the importance of maintaining proper body weight and composition particularly for females. Next I wanted to see the results of obesity on the organs.

I went to the living healthy 360 website and found out the following:

1. The pancreas must work much harder to meet the increased demand for insulin in obese people. If not taken seriously, the overload eventually can cause a complete shutdown of insulin secretion, which in turn, will develop into diabetes.

2. A person with a higher fat percentage will have a higher risk for hypertension and "bad" cholesterol. This increases the risk for heart disease as well as congestive heart failure. I was amazed to find out that obesity causes non alcoholic fatty liver disease, that can lead to complete liver failure. I already put my poor liver through enough, particularly because I live near a college bar (shout out to Effins Pub on El Cajon Blvd, what's up Luke Carlsen!! WOOOO!! Keep them Jamos comin, son).

3. Lung function is affected by obesity and capacity is reduced because of increased demand in oxygen. Anyone that has ever seen me climbing the stairs at work can attest to this.
4. Obesity is a key factor in erectile dysfunction and leads to decreased libido and energy levels.

Whoa. Let's not get crazy.

Here's a picture of my boss, Katrina, CEO of www.fitnessinked.com to cleanse the palette, so to speak.

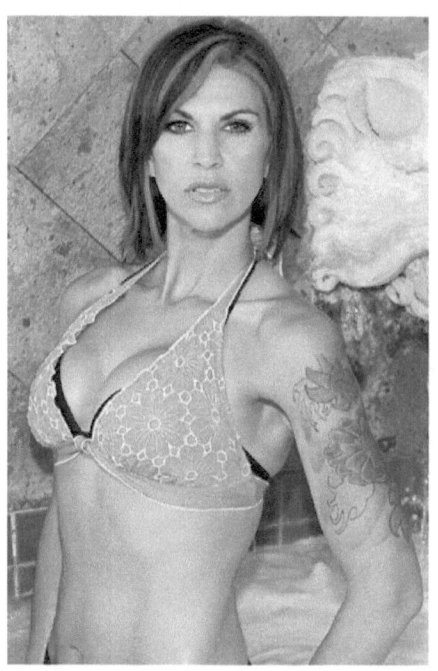

Thanks for helping, Kat. Now back to this awful subject. Anything that is going to affect my ability as a Viking in the bedroom should be taken seriously. God knows I wasn't blessed with looks, charm, or decency. At the very least, I want to be able to enjoy consensual relations with women of

questionable virtue and hopefully, bad
eyesight.

Skinny Dragon Plan- Basic

8. Confidence and Perception

I have been both a large guy and a very fit guy. The difference in how people treated me was noticeable. Society rewards the fit and attractive. I'm sorry to be the one to break it to you and for many, it's not exactly breaking news, but attractive people get hired more, make more money, and have more opportunities in life.

Don't believe me? Ask Victoria Silverstedt. Every picture I have ever seen of her is on a yacht in a bikini. I don't even think she can read. Do you really think these billionaires are saying, "Hey, call Vicky, we need someone to discuss international monetary policy and an exit strategy for Afghanistan."

According to Daniel Hamermesh, a professor at UT in Austin, attractive people are likely to earn 3 to 4 percent more than someone with below average looks (DAMN YOU, RYAN REYNOLDS). That doesn't seem like a lot but over a lifetime? Its about 230,000 dollars.

A study conducted in Europe attempted to find out if attractive people get more job opportunities. They sent out 10000 resumes with photos. The findings were clear. 54% of attractive women got a callback for an interview. Unattractive women got a 7% callback rate. Attractive men had a 47% callback rate, whereas unattractive men had a 26% callback rate.

Chris Christie, the governor of New Jersey, is a very smart, very successful man. Throughout his political career, he has been besieged by the media about his weight. He has been a large person for the majority of his life, and it has affected public perception of him.

It has been suggested that his chances for a presidential bid wouldn't be taken seriously because of his weight and possible future health issues. He recently got lap band surgery, which I think is a good step for his lifestyle (I don't condone surgery for every case, but for chronically obese people, I think it can save lives as a last resort).

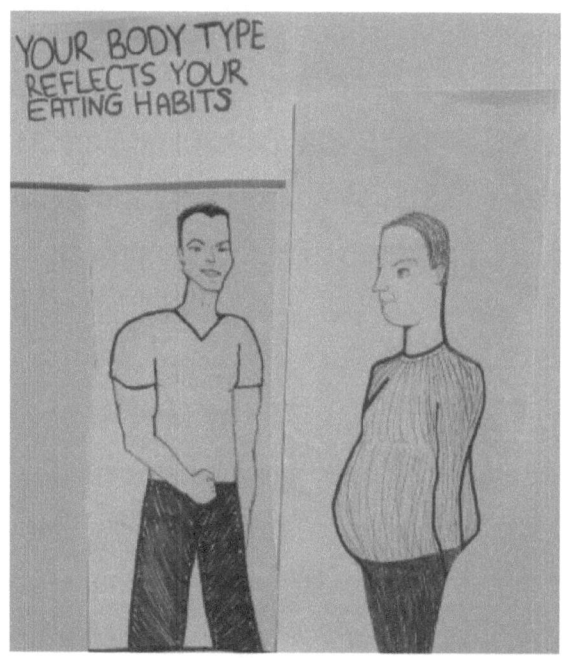

Confidence is going to play a very big part in your lives. Some of you have never known what it is like to have it. It's intoxicating. It can be used for a better life, better relationships, and better opportunities. That is why I wrote this book. When you look in the mirror and you have gotten to your optimal point of attraction, NOT society's, you will experience a change in life. I have been there a few times and it's always great.

I don't pretend that there is some magical weight or size that will fit every body type. _But I DO know that if you adapt Skinny Dragon to your life, you can find the one that works for you_. I would strongly encourage you to highlight the previous sentence and really think about what that means. Stop worrying about trying to look like an anorexic Hollywood actress or a fashion model.

If you're a girl, most guys I know are happy if you can cook a steak and look good most of the time. If you're a guy, most girls just like you to be able to talk to them and want you to have nice arms and some stubble on your face. Seriously, I'm like a 5 (maybe a 7 if you are out drinking tequila with your girlfriends and I've been working out), and I have dated some HOT women. Its all because I am confident, and fun. Use this plan to better yourself, the ensuing results will have a ripple effect of awesomeness.

And with that, here
is.................................the Skinny Dragon
Plan:

9. How the Plan Works/WHY the plan works

The Skinny Dragon Plan is a hybrid of several diets plus the end result of many articles I have read. Like Frankenstein's monster, it is a piece of this, and a piece of that, but the end result is that IT WORKS.

The technical description is as follows: *"The Skinny Dragon Plan is a semi-ketogenic, portion control meal allocation system that reduces the harmful intake of excessive white flour, while maximizing the beneficial effects of fruits, nuts, lean meats, and vegetables."*

The Rob version of that statement? "You eat less shitty food, and dump a bunch of weight. Then you start getting confident, buying new clothes, and cool people will want to hook up with you." Strangely enough, my editor strongly suggests that I don't use this phraseology on the marketing materials.

The way I wrote the plan had the following goals:

1. Let you be able to eat throughout the day without being hungry.

2. Expose you to new foods that you may have never tried.

3. Let you enjoy some reward foods while encouraging better habits about food.

4. Have several factors working in your favor to maximize fat loss.

The plan itself calls for you to choose three weeks, starting on a Sunday. You will fast for the first night (this will be explained in detail later), and then start taking your food with you in a cooler, using Tupperware. I made this plan easy and gave direct steps for you to follow. Then I made a list of foods you SHOULD eat, and in what portions. I also included a list of forbidden foods.

I also tell you to get off your ass, and exercise at least three times a week. Ride a bike, run, walk with the kids, Zumba, whatever, but you need to be active. Don't try to tell me you are too busy. I wake up at 4am some mornings to run. No excuses, remember?

The plan itself is quite ingenious and by implementing it, you have a MUCH higher chance of long term success, because you aren't dieting, you are creating a new system of meal planning. I have created a plan that reduces your chance of engaging in bad food choices.

Once you engage in the Skinny Dragon Plan you are doing the following:

1. Not eating fast food.

2. Not drinking soda

3. Not causing excess damage to your organs with white flour

4. Eating healthy, SMALL meals

5. Engaging in more exercise

6. Cutting your excess sodium intake

7. Greatly increasing your intake of vegetables

8. Eliminating fried foods from your diet

9. Not being tempted to do a 3000 calorie lunch with coworkers

Think about last month alone. How many times did you engage in some items from this list? I calculated how much I DIDNT consume in two weeks by following the plan and not eating with coworkers, and it was about 13000 calories. IN TWO WEEKS.

10. Other Plans

There are a lot of plans out there. I think that you should be well informed and choose one that is right for your lifestyle. Some of the most popular diets I researched were:

- South Beach
- Paleo
- Atkins
- The Zone
- Caveman Diet

As far as dieting books go, I would STRONGLY recommend the aforementioned *4 Hour Body* and *Man 2.0: Engineering the Alpha*. Both books are very similar and even reference each other. Tim Ferriss is a genius and I use several of his methods.

You may be wondering why I am telling you about potential competitors in my field. My job is to find what's right for YOU. By offering the most effective, and fastest methods of weight loss, I want to enable you to maximize your results, whether you use Skinny Dragon, Paleo, or Jenny Craig. Your happiness is my reward.

The difference between Skinny Dragon and other plans is the portion management component. By packing your own food every day, and controlling your portion size, you are limiting your consumption to what is on your plan, not being at the mercy of vending machines, restaurants, fast food, and other sources of an early death.

11. The Foods

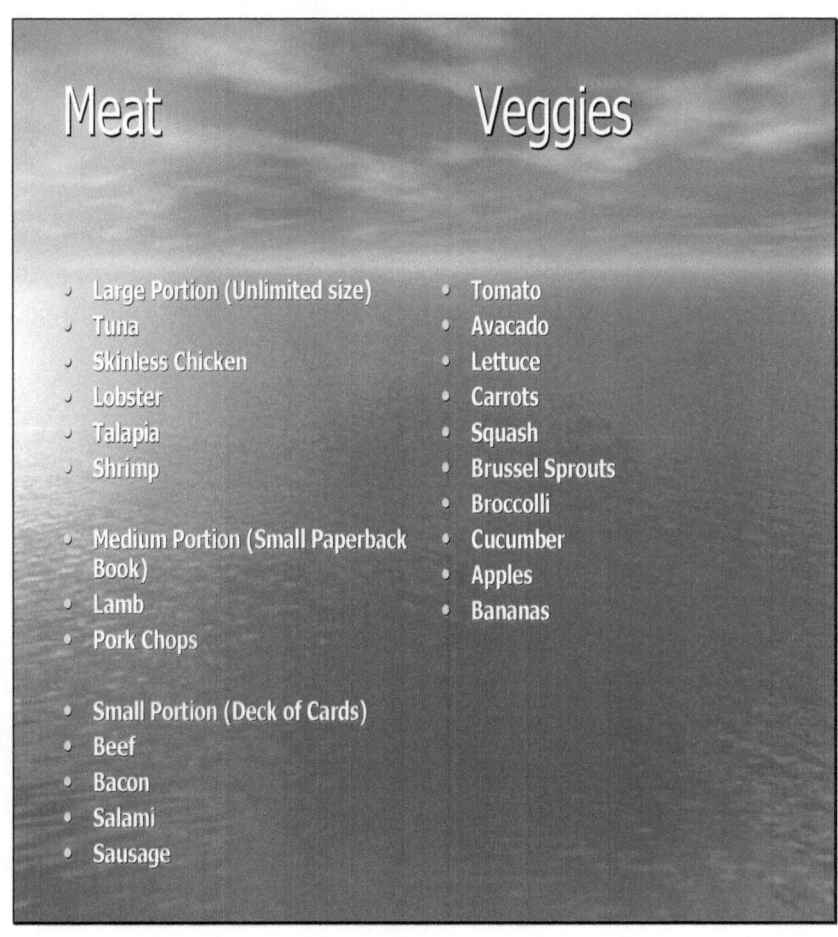

Meat

- Large Portion (Unlimited size)
- Tuna
- Skinless Chicken
- Lobster
- Talapia
- Shrimp

- Medium Portion (Small Paperback Book)
- Lamb
- Pork Chops

- Small Portion (Deck of Cards)
- Beef
- Bacon
- Salami
- Sausage

Veggies

- Tomato
- Avacado
- Lettuce
- Carrots
- Squash
- Brussel Sprouts
- Broccolli
- Cucumber
- Apples
- Bananas

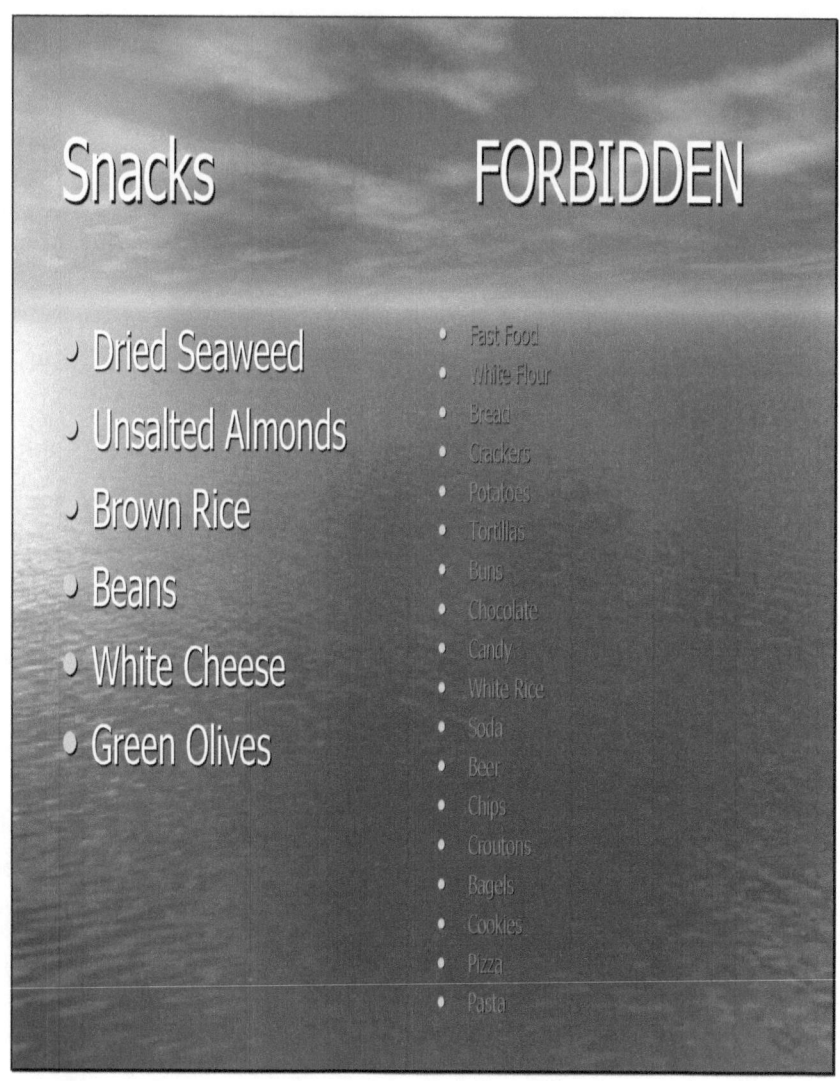

Snacks

FORBIDDEN

- Dried Seaweed
- Unsalted Almonds
- Brown Rice
- Beans
- White Cheese
- Green Olives

- Fast Food
- White Flour
- Bread
- Crackers
- Potatoes
- Tortillas
- Buns
- Chocolate
- Candy
- White Rice
- Soda
- Beer
- Chips
- Croutons
- Bagels
- Cookies
- Pizza
- Pasta

12. The Habits

1. I strongly suggest cooking for the week on Sunday night. Chop your veggies, cook a large quantity of meat, make chili in the crockpot. If you have kids, you can make their lunches.

2. Prepare for unexpected events. Always take a little extra. Just because you have more food doesn't mean you will overeat. An extra Ziploc baggie of carrots and celery might help you avoid a trip through the drive through.

3. Buy a freezer cold pack to go in your cooler. These things are GREAT for keeping your cooler cold for meats and cheeses.

4. The time to have your food ready is the NIGHT before, not the day of. You have enough chaos in the morning. Prep work saves you time. Every morning I grab my cooler, remove six Tupperware dishes from the fridge and that's it. All day meal plan is ready.

5. Starting on the second Sunday of the plan, you get a cheat day. Don't use this as an excuse to lose your mind. Eat the foods you

have avoided in small quantities. Cheat days
exist as a reward, not an excuse.

13. The Plan

The Skinny Dragon Plan

INTRO

First of all, congratulations. Trying something new like this is a great step in courage. You obviously want a change and I am grateful you are going to trust me with your most valuable possessions: your body and health. I have been a heavy/round guy for a lot of my life. Even though I worked out a lot in the military, I had no grasp of nutrition. Once I started learning,around 31 years old, I dabbled in Atkins and along with a lot of running, got down to a good weight. Fast forward a few years, and I started reading more books about fitness and nutrition, specifically, the five most popular diet books in the country. I grabbed an idea here, a concept there, and came up with what I feel is a powerful weapon to help you control your weight and to keep you healthy, happy, and most of all full of confidence.

HOW IT WORKS

The Skinny Dragon plan creates a multi-tiered attack to literally attack food the minute you eat it. Your body will start craving food in order to digest and absorb it faster. Once you have been on the Plan for about 12 days, ketosis kicks in and your body will literally just start eating fat from the inside. I lost fat from my muffin top, my butt, and my face got skinnier. The hardest part is getting to day 12 intact. You will start with a basic intermittent fast in order to prime your body for its new intake process. Then you will follow the basic rules outlined and eat only the foods that are on the SDP list. If you can make it to day 14, you earn a cheat day where you get to eat anything you want!! Then you do an intermittent fast, and the process starts over.

THE RULES

1. Follow the plan! If you cheat, accept it, and take steps to not cheat again.

2. Ketosis is like a race track broken into 12 sections (days of eating right). If you consume anything with white flour, you go right back to the starting line. You know what's at the finish line? CHEAT DAY. Don't be weak. Stick it out.

3. Don't tell anyone you are doing this. You know why? Your friends are stupid. You don't need any more advice from people that think the Kardashians are important or that 2Chainz is talented. Unless your friend has a Master's in Nutrition, or is a Navy SEAL, don't give up any info. Let them wonder how you got thinner in three weeks.

4. This plan will run for three weeks. Start on a Sunday.

COMMON TERMS

Ketosis- condition in which the liver starts an internal consumption of fat because of reduced intake of carbohydrates. Safely used since the 1930s to treat obesity.

Intermittent Fasting- Limiting food intake to 8 hours a day and not eating for 16 hours. This has a few benefits, such as restructuring your hormones so that more fat is burned and limiting your risk of certain diseases. The first day you do this, your food will taste five times better.

CHEATING

Cheating can be any of the following:
*eating during an intermittent fast
*eating flour
*eating anything on the forbidden list
*not doing your three sessions of exercise in a week

THE PROCESS

Review the food list carefully. Buy whatever items you want to eat during the diet that are on the recommended list. Cook and prepare your food for the week and pack your food in your Tupperware. The Sunday you start, eat like a pig. Literally, anything. At 8pm, you start your fast. You completely stop eating except for coffee, tea, or gum. Weigh yourself and write it down.

Monday the next day. You will take your cooler and your meals to work with you. You will NOT EAT until noon. (I want to be clear, YOU DO NOT EAT FROM 8PM SUNDAY TO NOON MONDAY). Once noon rolls around, you'll be very hungry. Dig in. You earned it.

For the rest of the week, just try to eat four small meals a day. Each meal should be small to medium sized and contain a meat, veggie(s), and a small amount of a fat (cheese, butter). Snacks are ok in small portions. I also gave you suggested portion size in relation to the fat content of the meats. Try to stop eating at 8pm, but you don't have to fast. You can have breakfast.

You will also need to incorporate exercise into your plan. I suggest either a 45 minute walk or a 30 minute run, minimum of three times a week.

This plan is just built to shrink fat. If you want to tone as well, check out my blog and do the exercises listed. Google Blue Dragon Enterprises Blog and look for the article called Blue Dragon Diet. There are exercises to shape your butt, abs, and chest.

The next fast will be the next Sunday. Same hours. If you can make it to the third Sunday (2 full weeks) with no flour, you can consider it a cheat day. ANYTHING GOES. Just stop eating at 8pm. Between the 2nd and 3rd week, you should see your first ketosis related drop in weight. It's the greatest moment you will remember. After the third week, you're done. Weigh yourself and send me the result.

3 Good Recipes That Are Safe and Healthy

Tomato Caprese

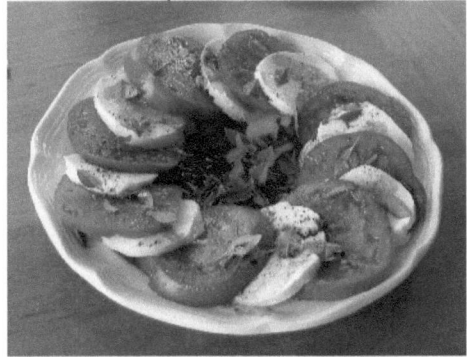

Tomato
Jack or Mozzarella
Italian Dressing
Parsley
Pepper

Turkey Chili

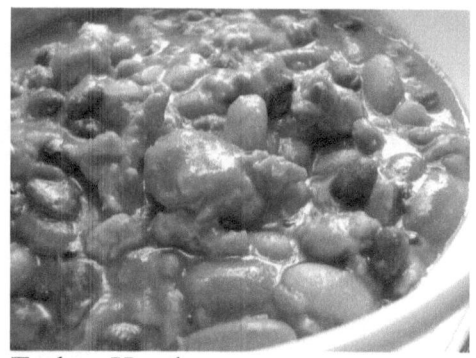

Turkey Hamburger
Black Beans
Garlic
Peppers
Onion

Brussel Sprouts and Bacon

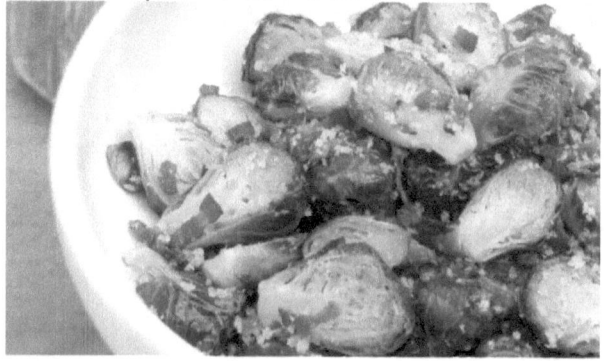

Brussel Sprouts
Bacon
Parmesan
Butter

EXTRA SNEAKY TIPS

*If you are having a BAD day, where you feel like you are starving, have one apple, a handful of almonds, and five cubes of white cheese. It will stave your hunger and you can feel good about sticking to your plan.

*Try new veggies. I have been eating buttered brussel sprouts, squash, and sliced bell peppers. It looks amazing and tastes great.

*Lemon pepper is excellent on fish and a great substitute for salt.

Skinny Dragon Plan- Basic

14. 30 Day Assessment and Adjustment

At 30 days, you should do an assessment and see how you have changed. The first thing people do is check the scale. I don't agree with this. If you lift weights while doing this plan, you will get heavier, but not fatter. This still isn't indicative of fitness or better health, it just means you have more mass. The best way to see if there is a change is to gauge against the following:

1. Is your face skinnier, and more defined?
2. Have you lost weight in fat accumulation areas like double chin, sides, belly?
3. Do your clothes fit better?
4. Do a significantly higher amount of people check you out? (I am dead serious on this one. If you look in the mirror, LIKE what you see, others will too. You can call me an idiot, but I have seen this countless times).
5. Are you able to run, exercise, or do cardio with more ease?

You should be able to see changes. You should also notice that people are treating you better, nicer, and are more likely to want to be around you. You should examine how you have felt, and if the foods you selected need tweaking. I still adjust the diet according to how much exercise I am doing. 8 mile run? More peanut butter and a banana. No exercise? Smaller portions, and lighter meats. The beauty of the plan is it's versatility.

And with that, the book is finished. I hope it helps you develop a new lifestyle of health, confidence, and mental well being. Do you have a success story to share? Email me at robleegarcia@yahoo.com. Id love to congratulate you.

Sincerely,
Dr. Rob Garcia

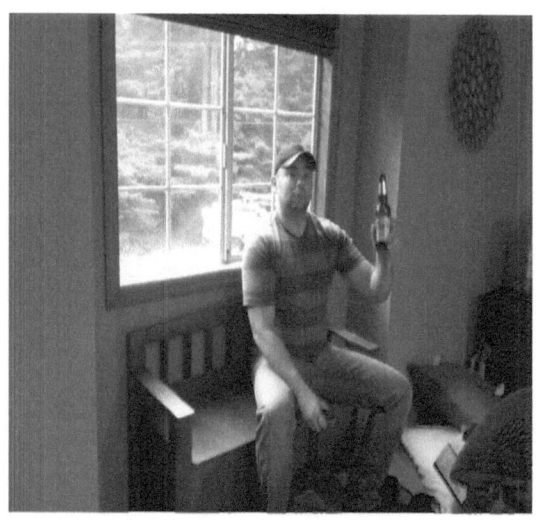

"I have been both of these guys. Weight management is not easy, but pays huge dividends" - Dr. Rob Garcia

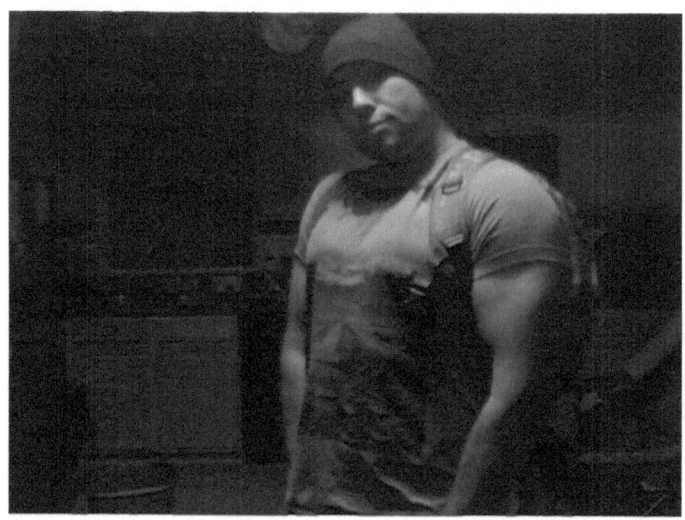